Let's Hack Male Infertility
Use 3 Lifestyle Choices to Reduce Your Oxidative Stress and Improve Your Sperm

Peter Stroot

Let's Hack Male Infertility by Peter Stroot

www.hemagnosis.com

© 2018 Peter Stroot

Visit the author's website at http://hemagnosis.com/blog/wp/.

Disclaimer

This book provides information that should not take the place of medical advice. I encourage you to talk to your healthcare providers (doctor, registered dietitian, pharmacist, etc.) about your interest in, questions about, or use of new fitness activities, food items, and dietary supplements and what may be best for your overall health. Any mention in this book of a specific product or service, or recommendation from an organization or professional society, does not represent an endorsement by the author of that product, service, or expert advice.

Table of Contents

Introduction 4

    Oxidative Stress is a Wide-Spread Problem...........................4

    Healthy weight does not mean healthy Oxidative Stress level 5

    Oxidative Stress is Very Expensive 6

    Hack it!...7

What is Oxidative Stress? 8

    Beware of Two Vices! 8

    What causes BLOS?..9

Hack Strategy Outline 11

Hack Equipment & Supplies..12

Review your Current Lifestyle Choices 14

      Dosage Warning...17

Organize Your Hack Strategy...18

Record Your Observations 21

      MyFitnessPal is a Free Phone App To Help Organize Your Hack...........22

Start Hacking!..26

Share Your Hack Results...26

Conclusion...27

Additional Information..28

    Review My Book..28

    BLOS World™ Store...28

    BLOS Research 28

Introduction

Male infertility is a big problem in Western Countries. There are multiple theories on the cause, but Blood Oxidative Stress (BLOS) is the only theory that could explain the bulk of it. BLOS is widespread with more than 2/3 of adult Americans thought to suffer from it. The rise of the Western Diet and the increase of male infertility rates follow similar trends. In vitro fertilization (IVF) is a popular, yet expensive solution to the problem of infertility. IVF costs about $15,000 per cycle with many couples requiring multiple cycles for success. However, about 60% of infertility problems are attributed to unhealthy men. Clearly, diet and fitness (lifestyle choices) may be the primary cause of the infertility problems of many couples. So, improving the health of men with respect to BLOS may be an inexpensive solution to the infertility problem. Direct measurement of Oxidative Stress could be used as a tool to evaluate a man's lifestyle choices with the goal of getting healthier and consequently improving the health of his sperm.

Oxidative Stress is a Wide-Spread Problem

Oxidative Stress is the mysterious condition that seems to be affecting everyone. Every week, new links are reported between Oxidative Stress and health problems. Long-term, elevated Oxidative Stress should be considered an Asymptomatic Disease like Cardiovascular and Alzheimer's Diseases. Over time, elevated Oxidative Stress may manifest in several different health problems that may include Cardiovascular Disease, Obesity, Type 2 Diabetes, and more. Despite decades of medical research conducted by thousands of researchers, a common genetic basis (i.e., mutation) for these health problems has not been discovered. At best, I expect that genetic mutations may play a role in the array and severity of symptoms. It's also well known that Oxidative Stress causes DNA damage, which is one of the principal means for developing Cancer. So, long-term, elevated Oxidative Stress increases your risk for developing Cancers. With all the evidence piling up, it's a good idea to learn more about Oxidative Stress and how to reduce if for the rest of your life. One of the side benefits of this

Hack is that your health should be improved and hopefully you'll stick to your new lifestyle choices for the rest of your life!

If you think that you're safe, because your weight is normal, then consider the following. Oxidative Stress depletes your own antioxidant protection, sodium sulfide (NaHS), which causes Hypertension. A simple model (**Figure 1**) links plasma NaHS concentration to Oxidative Stress level. The greater the Oxidative Stress level, the lower the NaHS concentration. Healthy individuals have very low levels of Oxidative Stress, while more severe health problems are associated with much higher levels of Oxidative Stress. Being Overweight or afflicted by Type 2 Diabetes is an indication of high Oxidative Stress. **While normal weight doesn't mean that you're necessarily healthy with respect to Oxidative Stress. It also doesn't mean that your Sperm are healthy.** The Oxidative Stress level for Normal Weight have a wide range. The only way to be sure that you're healthy is to measure your own Oxidative Stress level. The purple arrows provide guidance on the Oxidative Stress level when Pre-Diabetes and Atherosclerosis are triggered. The large blue arrow simply implies that greater Oxidative Stress level increases the risk of Cancer. If you think that you're healthy, then you should measure your weight <u>and</u> your Oxidative Stress level. If you're overweight or in worse health, then you're probably suffering from high Oxidative Stress. Will reducing and managing your Oxidative Stress improve your health? It's clear that maintaining your weight doesn't always work based on the normal weight people that develop severe health problems. Could long-term, elevated Oxidative Stress be the cause? Is there any alternative explanation?

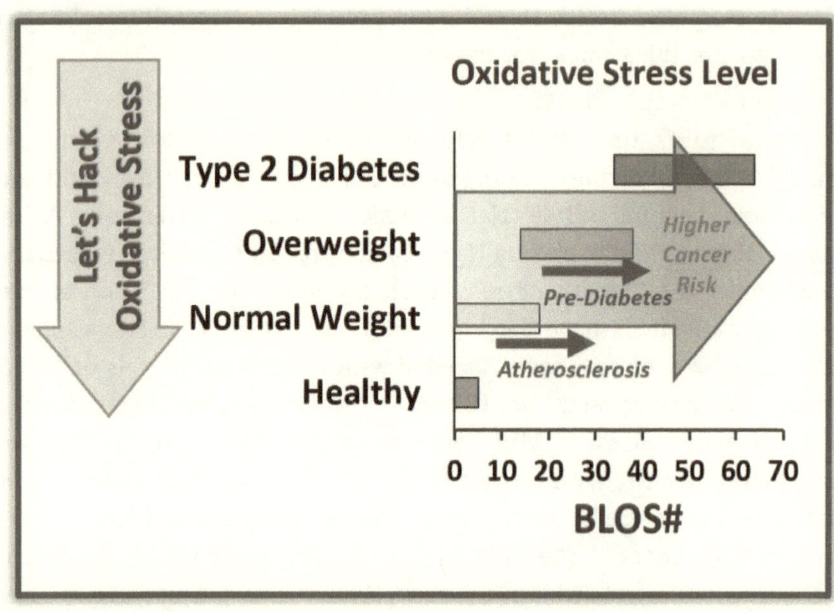

Figure 1 Relationship between Oxidative Stress Level and Health State

Oxidative Stress is Very Expensive

The large number of people suffering from long-term, elevated Oxidative Stress is costing a lot of money in healthcare. The sum of the percent of adult Americans that are either Overweight or Obese is more than 2/3 of adult Americans[1]. About 100 million adult Americans suffer from Prediabetes or Type 2 Diabetes[2]. Using available statistics from the CDC, it is estimated that the USA spends over $800B/year in healthcare costs that may be attributed to elevated Oxidative Stress. The chart above (**Figure 1**) should be hopeful to many folks suffering from poor health, since it implies that a reduction in Oxidative Stress may reverse some health conditions. Dietary changes are effective in reversing Type 2 Diabetes, although the true reason may not be excessive dietary carbohydrates, but elevated Oxidative Stress. Someday (or decade?), medical researchers will finally answer this question, but you don't need to

---

[1] https://www.cdc.gov/nchs/fastats/obesity-overweight.htm

[2] https://www.cdc.gov/media/releases/2017/p0718-diabetes-report.html

wait for their answer. Could lower Oxidative Stress improve or reverse other health conditions that have taken years or decades to progress? Caution would be prudent, since it may take some time for your body to recover. At the very least, lower Oxidative Stress may delay or prevent the onset of advanced symptoms of some of these health conditions. If the management of Oxidative Stress can prevent the advancement of many health problems, then we will reduce healthcare costs and make healthcare more affordable. There are more potential benefits including longer life expectancy, better quality of life, higher productivity, and more.

This isn't just a problem for the USA, Europe and many countries that have adopted the Western Diet have similar numbers. Just read the news on the growing number of people that are Obese or diagnosed with Type 2 Diabetes. Elevated Oxidative Stress is also impacting our children. Is your child's school lunch program causing Oxidative Stress? How about the restaurant industry? Are they selling you food that is causing Oxidative Stress? Don't worry, I'm sure medical researchers and government regulators have a firm grasp on the situation and can provide sound advice on Oxidative Stress. (You're laughing, aren't you?) If you don't have a few decades to wait for the definitive answer from these experts, then you'll need to "take the bull by the horns" and learn more about Oxidative Stress and how lifestyle choices may help you manage it.

Hack it!

Humans have faced difficult problems in the past and solved some of them in a creative, empirical approach affectionately known as "hacking." It starts with constructing a simple model of the problem and then one attempts to change inputs or conditions to change the output. You're testing your own hypothesis on whether your model is accurate. In this case, your body is the "black box" that you're hacking. You make observations after making changes to the input or conditions and learn. You keep what works and discard what doesn't work. So, with Oxidative Stress, your only hope going forward is do what humans do best: If you can Track It, then you can Hack It! Let's start with learning more about Oxidative Stress.

What is Oxidative Stress?

Despite over 200,000 research articles on Oxidative Stress, there is little information on how to measure Oxidative Stress. Let's start with what we do know about Oxidative Stress. In general, Oxidative Stress is when cells generate high levels of reactive oxygen species or ROS, which oxidizes chemical compounds non-discriminately. The oxidation of these biomolecules can be measured in blood and urine samples, while ROS can also be measured directly in blood and breath. There are two sources of Oxidative Stress in humans (and other mammals): General and Blood. General Oxidative Stress is based on observations of pure tissue cultures under controlled conditions, which usually involves providing the tissue culture with excessive substrate (ex. Glucose). These simple experiments have led to more recent research that evaluates the role of carbohydrate rich diets in the generation of Oxidative Stress in lab animals. However, there is no method to identify which type of tissue is responsible for the bulk of the General Oxidative Stress. In contrast, Blood Oxidative Stress or BLOS was reported and a flow cytometry method was used to directly measure the percent of white blood cells and platelets that generated high levels of ROS (that's the BLOS# in **Figure 1**). In addition, this research article suggests that BLOS is the primary source of Oxidative Stress afflicting humans. Primary in this context means that General Oxidative Stress is not as important as BLOS. A major difference in the two types of Oxidative Stress lies in their mode of generation. General Oxidative Stress is thought to be a function of the substrate (ex. Glucose) concentration, so it is a short-term response (a few hours) that occurs after eating. In contrast, BLOS is continuous and is only a function of the percent of blood cells induced to generate ROS and the metabolic rate of the blood cells.

Beware of Two Vices!

There are two types of General Oxidative Stress associated with two popular vices: smoking and alcohol consumption. Smoking and alcohol consumption cause General Oxidative Stress in the lungs and liver, respectively. If you have any hope of Hacking Oxidative Stress, then you'll need to get a handle on these vices.

What causes BLOS?

There is only one mechanistic model (i.e., hypothesis) for BLOS, which I proposed a few years ago. Blood cells are induced to generate ROS from the consumption of high amounts of inorganic sulfur in the Western Diet. Sulfate reducing bacteria (SRB) in the large intestine increase in numbers with a diet rich in inorganic sulfur, which will eventually result in short periods (i.e., minutes) of ultra-exogenous sulfide formation (USF). This USF impacts the blood cells passing through the ascending colon and the elevated blood sulfide concentration induces these blood cells to start generating ROS to counteract the high concentration of blood sulfide. My research article provided several experiments that could be tested to evaluate my hypothesis. I'm not holding my breath waiting for Academics to conduct these experiments and neither should you. This USF reaction may be your body's built-in defense system to protect itself against a wound infection that is being triggered in a stealth way in your large intestine (my follow up research article). Diet induced BLOS may be your body trying to fight off a non-existent wound infection. In other words, your "black box" has a built-in defense system for one environmental insult (wound on your body poorly protected by clothing resulting in an infection of multiple bacteria), but it is being triggered by a modern environmental insult (Western Diet) in a part of your body that is difficult to monitor.

One strategy to manage BLOS may be to simply change your diet and prevent USF. Diets that reduce the amount of sulfur compounds reaching the large intestine may be effective in reducing USF. Are there other ways to combat Oxidative Stress? **Antioxidants** are chemical compounds that neutralize ROS compounds. There are a multitude of supplements and food items that purport to be rich in antioxidants, but do they work? Antioxidants are compounds that react with ROS to neutralize it. Antioxidants come in many forms from individual compounds synthesized in a laboratory to a fruit extract or even dehydrated fruit. These compounds are brought together into a "formula", which is either encapsulated or pressed into a pill. The supplement can also be prepared in such a way to make it "sustained release" or "slow release", which means that the capsule will slowly dissolve in the small intestine and not rapidly in the stomach. BLOS is continuous, so a sustained release supplement may be more effective compared to supplement that provides a spike of antioxidant. This fact may also be the reason that so many experiments with antioxidants provide no improvement in Oxidative Stress (and health).

With more complete knowledge that BLOS is the primary source of Oxidative Stress that needs to be managed, the Hack of Oxidative Stress may be possible. Three lifestyle choices are available for your Hack Strategy.   Using one of the popular diets that limit your processed carbohydrates may be effective in reducing your consumption of inorganic sulfur, since many food items with processed have food preservatives and additives containing inorganic sulfur. So, stick to one of these popular diets or just make an effort to reduce processed carbohydrates in your diet (and read those food labels!). The addition of effective fitness activity may also help your body generate nitric oxide and stimulate the production of endogenous (made by you) sodium sulfide, your body's own antioxidant. The addition of an effective antioxidant supplement like Vitamin E and/or Vitamin C may help reduce your Oxidative Stress. These three lifestyle choices can be brought together into an effective strategy to Hack Male Infertility.

Hack Strategy Outline

Here's a 6-step outline of the strategy for your personal Hack of Male Infertility.

1. Review current lifestyle choices that may be contributing to Oxidative Stress.

2. Organize your Hack to evaluate new lifestyle choices that may reduce your Oxidative Stress.

3. Record your observations before and after you start your Hack.

4. Review your observations to determine whether your new lifestyle choices reduced your Oxidative Stress.

5. Collect and analyze Sperm Count and Health after lowering Oxidative Stress.

6. Share your Hack results.

Hack Equipment & Supplies

For this Hack (**Figure 2**), two products are essential including the Urine Oxidative Stress Test Kit and the YO Home Sperm Test. There are many optional products that also may be useful for this Hack including Fitness Equipment, Diet Book, and Antioxidant Supplements. Check the **BLOS World™ Store** for more information on these products.

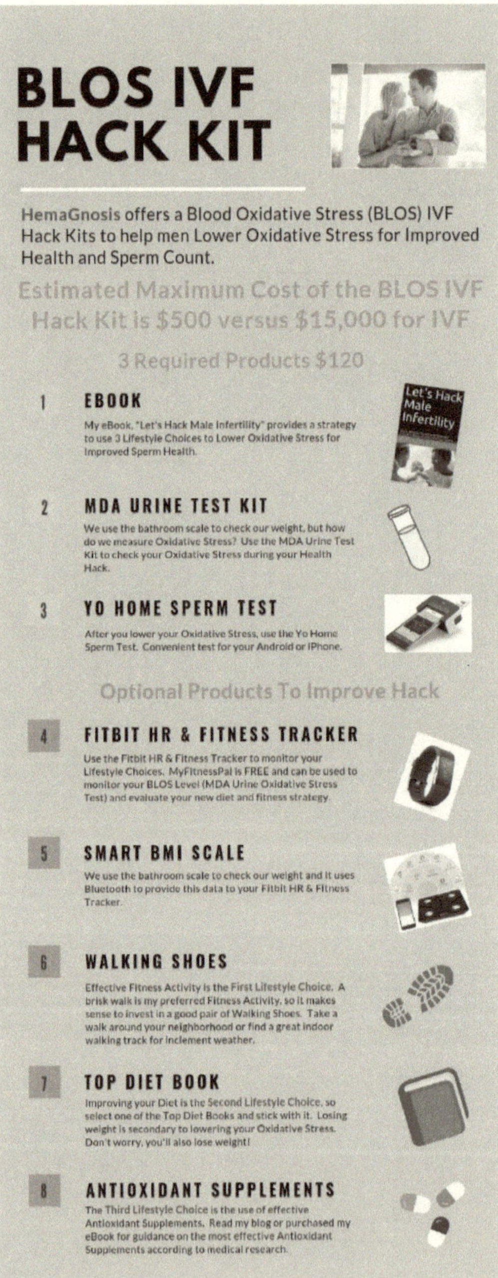

Figure 2 Hack Male Infertility Infographic with Essential and Optional Products

Review your Current Lifestyle Choices

Before getting started with formulating your Oxidative Stress Hack Strategy, you will need to be very honest about your current health state and lifestyle choices.

Current Health State

The most important measure of your current Health State may be your Oxidative Stress or BLOS Level. Your estimated BLOS Range is a function of your Diabetic State. Normal Diabetic State is defined by healthy blood glucose levels and corresponds to a BLOS Range of 0-20%. ***With respect to BLOS, a measured BLOS# value of less than 5% is considered Healthy.*** So, you may still be suffering from elevated BLOS, if you have a Normal Diabetic State. Pre-diabetes afflicts a large number of adult Americans and corresponds to an estimated BLOS Range of 15-40%. Type 2 Diabetics have a much greater estimated BLOS Range of 35-65%. If you're making Lifestyle changes including diet and fitness, then you want to measure your Urine Oxidative Stress level. This is the only way to ensure that your Lifestyle Choices are reducing Oxidative Stress.

In addition to measuring your current Oxidative Stress or BLOS level, you should measure your weight, resting blood pressure, and resting heart rate. Your weight measurement can be combined with your height to calculate your Body Mass Index (BMI). The BMI is another way to evaluate your current health status. Here's a good website that provides a free BMI calculator: https://www.webmd.com/diet/body-bmi-calculator You can track your weight and BMI by using a Smart BMI bathroom scale with Bluetooth, which can be linked directly to your Fitbit Fitness Tracker. The phone app MyFitnessPal can also be used to monitor your weight, BMI, and dietary choices. In addition, there is a way to modify this Free phone app to record your Urine Oxidative Stress measurements (**MyFitnessPal is a Free Phone App To Help Organize Your Hack**).

CAUTION: If you have a diagnosed health condition, then you should review any changes in your lifestyle choices with your physician. All the lifestyle choices may not be available to you, but you won't know until you meet with your physician to review your health and the three lifestyle choices.

If you're a smoker and/or drinker, then you should be very honest with yourself and accurately describe your habit. This Hack would be a great opportunity to reduce or eliminate these habits. I think it will be very difficult for a heavy smoker or drinker to Hack Oxidative Stress. Maybe you'll surprise me, but I doubt it.

Beyond vices, there are three primary lifestyle choices that influence Oxidative Stress, as shown in **Figure 3**: 1) Diet, 2) Fitness, and 3) Antioxidant   Supplements.

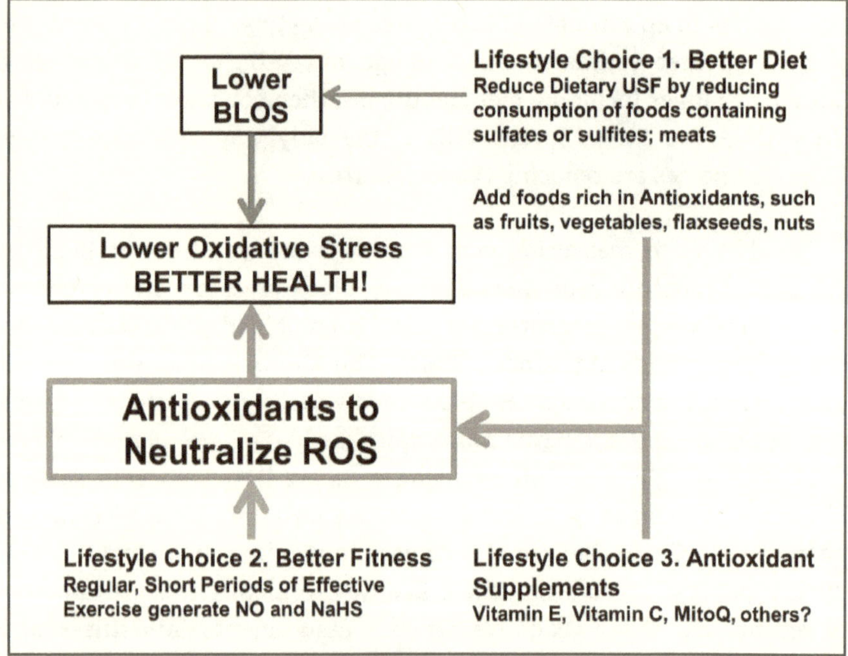

Figure 3 Three Lifestyle Choices Affect Oxidative Stress Level

Lifestyle Choice 1. Diet Do you follow an effective diet that maintains your weight? If not, then you should review some of the more popular diets out there and adopt one. Or you can simply make the effort to reduce the many processed carbohydrates that are the staple of the Western Diet. This alone should reduce the amount of inorganic sulfur that you consume, which may help reduce BLOS. A moderate reduction in protein, animal or vegetable, will also reduce the amount of organic sulfur (i.e., amino acids), which will also be helpful. SRB can grow on sulfur containing amino acids, but slowly. Diet is your most important weapon to fight Oxidative Stress, but fitness activity and antioxidant supplements are also available.

Lifestyle Choice 2. Fitness Do you exercise religiously? If not, then now is the time to try the simplest exercise available to just about everyone: walking. When done right, walking can get your heart rate up to the level that you'll need to signal to your body to start making nitric oxide or NO (helps with hypertension) and the production of endogenous sodium sulfide, an antioxidant that your body makes for free. Although this isn't enough NaHS to counter BLOS, every little bit helps, and the benefit of regular NO production shouldn't be dismissed.

Lifestyle Choice 3. Antioxidant Supplements Finally, you need to review your use of supplements, especially antioxidant supplements. If you're not using antioxidant supplements, then you'll be overwhelmed by the choices available at your local supermarket or pharmacy. It can be a bit daunting, but here's the key information that you'll need to know.

Vitamin E is probably the most effective antioxidant available. So, head to the store and purchase a bottle of high quality Vitamin E supplements or stop by the BLOS World Store and purchase one that I've identified as a great Vitamin E supplement through Amazon: https://amzn.to/2NW0edz. To my knowledge, a sustained release Vitamin E supplement is not available, which is probably due to the oily nature of this supplement. If one becomes commercially available, then I'll provide an update on my blog.

A recent research article that described the use of **Vitamin C** to treat sepsis demonstrates the importance of the supplement format.

Intravenous (IV) delivery of a cocktail that includes Vitamin C effectively reduces Oxidative Stress in sepsis patients leading to recovery. Although IV treatment with Vitamin C is gaining popularity in some Health Clubs in California, it is cost prohibitive. However, a sustained release Vitamin C supplement may be just as effective. If this approach interests you for your Hack, then carefully check the labels of the Vitamin C supplements at your favorite health food store, pharmacy, or pharmacy section of your grocery store. If you're having difficulty finding a high-quality Vitamin C supplement, then consider this one offered through Amazon: https://amzn.to/2xOeCKF.

Be aware that the research on antioxidants is rapidly advancing. Another recent report suggests that **MitoQ** may be very effective in reducing Oxidative Stress and should be investigated further before purchasing due to the rather steep price of about $2/day. However, if you're motivated to reduce Oxidative Stress, then you could purchase the MitoQ supplement through Amazon: https://amzn.to/2JV02V9

Dosage Warning

Resist the urge to use too much or too many different antioxidant supplements. Stick to the vendor's recommendation on the proper dosage. Wait to switch, increase, or add new antioxidant supplements for a few weeks to determine whether your Hack is effective. In the long-term, you want to determine the minimum dose of antioxidant supplement that will manage your Oxidative Stress. Why spend extra money on an antioxidant supplement that provides marginal improvement?

Organize Your Hack Strategy

To Hack Male Infertility, you're going to need to get organized. Based on your Current Lifestyle Choices, you will need to plan on adjusting at least one of your Current Lifestyle Choices that may be causing Oxidative Stress. ***Always consult with your physician before changing your diet, fitness routine, or supplements!***

Lifestyle Choice 1. Diet

For your dietary changes, record your current diet for at least 1 week before starting. If you're going to change your diet for your Hack, then be sure to review your dietary plan and purchase all of the food items that you'll need for at least the first week. Remove any food items that may tempt you and donate to a local food pantry. If you enjoy snacks at work, then you want to replace all those unhealthy snacks, too. Excessive dining out may also be counterproductive for your diet, unless you can be sure that you're making good menu decisions. Your best bet is to avoid restaurants and eat at home or pack a lunch. Give yourself a few weeks of a Spartan lifestyle to determine whether your Hack was successful. You can slowly increase your dining out in the future and use the Oxidative Stress test kit to determine whether it is problematic.

Lifestyle Choice 2. Fitness

The simplest equipment for improving your fitness are a good pair of walking shoes and a heart rate monitor. Identify a good walking route near your home. Test the walking route for any potential problems, such as aggressive dogs or hoodlums. You don't want to select a route with a lot of stoplights that will slow you down! If your neighborhood is a bit dicey, then consider your local mall or a park. Be sure to check the sidewalk or road surface before starting your Hack journey. You don't need to twist an ankle due an uneven sidewalk or potholes on the shoulder of the road that are on your walking route. Be sure to give yourself a total of one hour to complete your walk. It should take you about 15 minutes to increase your heart rate to an effective range (80% of the maximum for your age and gender but check with your physician for guidance). Once you've reached the target range for your heart rate, then you will want to maintain for 15-30 minutes. Allow about 15 minutes for cool down. For some folks, a weighted backpack may be needed to reach the target range. A blood pressure monitoring device and scale are optional, but they could provide more positive feedback. If walking in your neighborhood is not going to work for you, then consider alternatives, such as a local gym that has a treadmill or similar apparatus. Many gyms will offer a walking track, so do your homework and investigate. If you have a disability or physician's orders to not increase your fitness, then you'll still have two Lifestyle Choices available for your Hack.

Lifestyle Choice 3. Antioxidant Supplements

If your local health food store does not have your choice for antioxidant supplements, then order your antioxidant supplements well in advance to ensure that they're available for your Hack. Be sure that you have plenty of the supplement for the duration of your Hack. Pill organizers come in handy to ensure that you actually take your supplements every day. I keep my pill organizer near the bathroom sink to ensure that I see it every morning before I start the day.

Measure Oxidative Stress

Expensive, physician prescribed tests for measuring Oxidative Stress in blood are available, but unsuitable for this Hack due to the cost. Instead, purchase the Urine Oxidative Stress test kit (https://amzn.to/2zGBpti) in advance of your Hack. This kit is the only kit ($52.99/25 count) that is available to the public. This kit provides 25 test strips, so you may want to order a second kit for an extended Hack test. Another way to extend the use of this kit is to measure your Oxidative Stress every other day, which will give you a total of 50 days for your pre-Hack and Hack. Even better, get a friend to split the cost of the kit. Read all directions and use the kit to measure your own Oxidative Stress before your Hack. This kit provides a colorimetric strip that will provide the level of ROS in your urine as Minimal, Low, Medium, or High. **The goal is to reach the Minimal level of Oxidative Stress and maintain this level for a few weeks <u>before</u> evaluating your sperm.** Bear in mind that it takes 2-3 months for your sperm to fully mature in your body[3] . Lengthy exposure of your sperm to Oxidative Stress may be causing damage. So, you may want to wait 3 months after reducing your Oxidative Stress to evaluate your sperm. Keep to your own schedule on when you'll be measuring your Urine Oxidative Stress level. For some folks this will be in the morning after waking up, while others may prefer to test in the evening. Try not to vary your beverage consumption before and during the Hack, since this may influence your Hack (dilution or concentration of Oxidative Stress). The use of a supplement with B-vitamins may also alter the color of the test strip, so be sure to read the instructions carefully.

Evaluate Sperm Count and Health

A new DIY Sperm Evaluation Kit is now available for either Android (https://amzn.to/2QH3qXR) or iPhone (https://amzn.to/2xu3gur). This Kit is designed for two tests, so you will want to use the first test to evaluate your current Oxidative Stress level. After you have reduced your Oxidative Stress level for a few weeks, you will use this kit to evaluate the second sperm sample. You and your physician will be able to compare and evaluate your Male Infertility Hack.

---

[3] https://www.mensjournal.com/health-fitness/12-things-every-man-should-know-about-sperm-20151026/the-vagina-is-a-harsh-environment-for-sperm/

Record Your Observations

It is very important that you record all your measurements and other observations during your Hack. This Hack may take a few weeks before you notice an improvement in your Oxidative Stress level. There are two approaches for recording your observations: old school and smart tech.

The old school method for recording your observations is also the simplest and inexpensive way to record your Oxidative Stress Hacking observations. Simply use a notebook and pen. Be sure to organize your information by date like a diary. Don't rely on your memory!

If you have access to a word processor, such as Microsoft Word, then you can setup and record your observations. Just insert a table and organize it for your Hack. Here's how I organized my electronic notebook in Microsoft Word (**Figure 4**):

Date	Oxidative Stress Hack (OSH) Day	Urine Test	AntiOxidant	Fitness Strategy	Observations: record resting BP, weight, etc.
			Type: Dose: Type: Dose:	Type: Duration:	
	OSH Day -7		Yes or No	Yes or No	
	OSH Day -6		Yes or No	Yes or No	
	OSH Day -5		Yes or No	Yes or No	
	OSH Day -4		Yes or No	Yes or No	
	OSH Day -3		Yes or No	Yes or No	
	OSH Day -2		Yes or No	Yes or No	
	OSH Day -1		Yes or No	Yes or No	
	OSH Day 1		Yes or No	Yes or No	
	OSH Day 2		Yes or No	Yes or No	
	OSH Day 3		Yes or No	Yes or No	
	OSH Day 4		Yes or No	Yes or No	

Figure 4 Microsoft Word document used to Organize a Hack of Oxidative Stress

If you have trouble with preparing an electronic notebook for your Oxidative Stress Hack test, then send me an email to pgstroot@hemagnosis.com and I'll send you a free PDF, Microsoft Word, or Excel file that can be used to record your Oxidative Stress Hack. The PDF is a great option for folks that do not have Microsoft Office but have access to a printer. If you don't own a printer, then you can always contact your local library for assistance. Some local business, such as grocery stores, UPS, and FedEx, could also help you with printing out a simple PDF for a very low rate of a few pennies per sheet. Don't let your lack of software be the excuse for not Hacking Oxidative Stress! A pen and a few sheets of a paper will always work in a pinch.

MyFitnessPal is a Free Phone App To Help Organize Your Hack

You can use a Free Phone App, MyFitnessPal, with your Android or iPhone to help organize your hack. The great app can be used directly to record your dietary choices, weight, and more. You can record your Urine Oxidative Stress (BLOS) measurements, too.

Download the **MyFitnessPal** app (https://amzn.to/2DoV4Sa). Setup your profile and select MY HOME menu option on your MyFitnessPal homepage (**Figure 5**). Next, select the Check-In menu and you will see the following screen. In the Track Additional Measurements screen, you simply fill in the Description below Add Another Measurement. I entered BLOS, but you can add other measurements like Blood Sugar, A1C, and more.

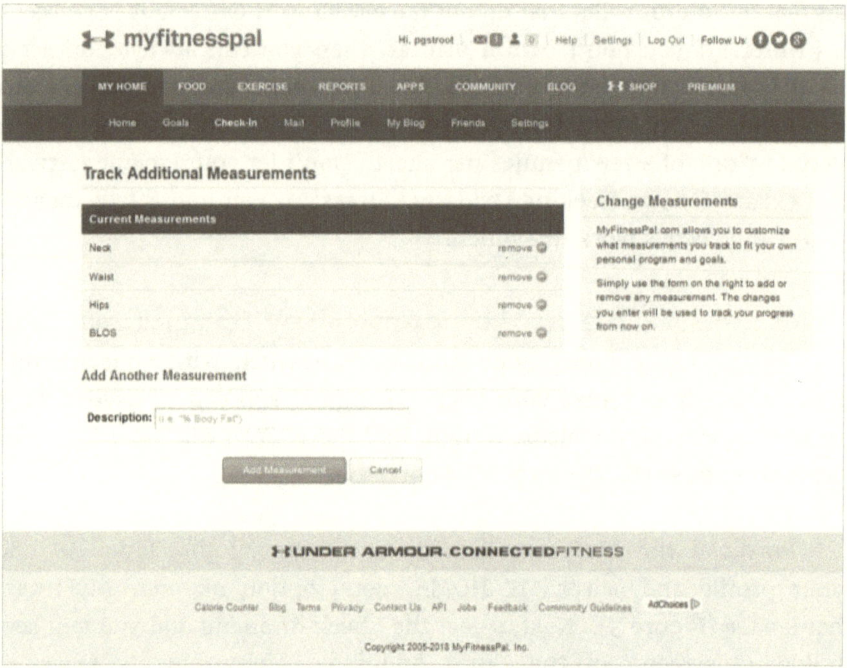

Figure 5 MyFitnessPal screen to Track Additional Measurements

For BLOS, you can use the Urine Oxidative Stress Test Kit to measure your Oxidative Stress. With this kit, you'll get a qualitative description of your BLOS or Oxidative Stress measurement. The color indicator strip will tell you if your BLOS level is Normal (5), Low (15), Medium (30), or High (45). These values are the best estimate of the BLOS# corresponding to these qualitative values of the Urine Oxidative Stress level. MyFitnessPal uses numbers and not values.

You can monitor or review your BLOS or other measurements by selecting the REPORTS menu option and then Charts sub-menu option (**Figure 6**). In the example below, I input BLOS of 15 for a Low BLOS measurement.

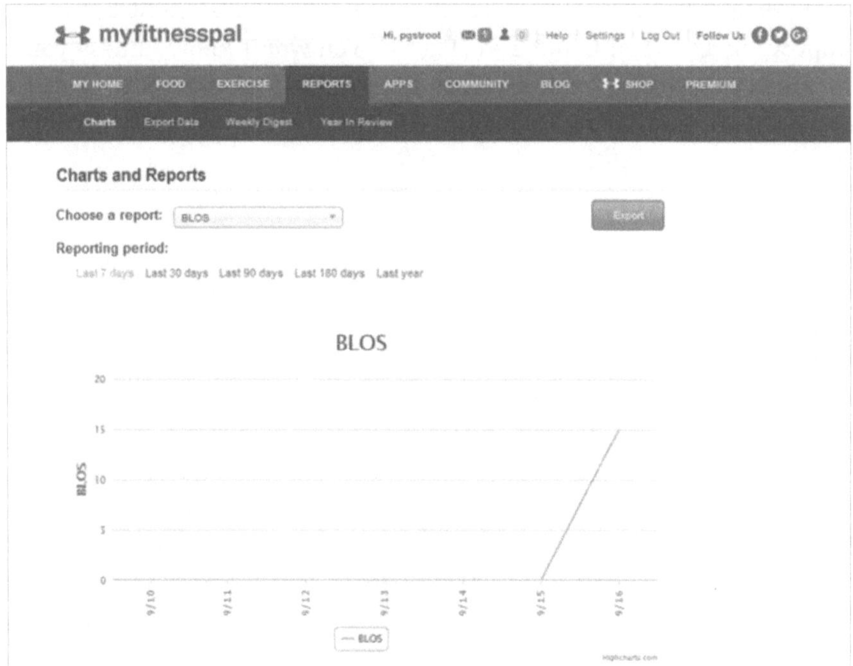

Figure 6 MyFitnessPal example of Chart used to track Urine Oxidative Stress (BLOS) measurement

MyFitnessPal could be a very useful tool for your Hack, since it will allow you to evaluate the impact of your lifestyle choices on your Oxidative Stress level. This approach may help you identify improper dietary choices, effective fitness, and more!

You need to record observations of your current Oxidative Stress status for one week <u>before</u> you start your Male Infertility Hack. In addition, you need to evaluate your Sperm Count and Health corresponding to your current Oxidative Stress status. It is very important to record this information, since you will need it to compare to your Oxidative Stress Hack observations. **How else will you know whether it worked?** This measurement is also very important, because it provides you with a direct measurement of your Oxidative Stress level attributed to your current lifestyle. So, take the time to measure your current Oxidative Stress before making the attempt to Hack it! Daily measurements would be ideal. Will your Male Infertility Hack strategy lower your Oxidative Stress level and improve your Sperm Count and Health? You won't know, unless you stick to your Hack strategy and measure the level of Oxidative Stress over time and evaluate your Sperm Count and Health.

Start Hacking!

At this point, you should have about 1 week of pre-Hack observations and you're now ready to start your Male Infertility Hack. While the primary method for evaluating the success of your Male Infertility Hack is the use of the Urine Strip Test, other measurements like resting blood pressure and weight may also shift (lower!) due to your lifestyle change, so be sure to be consistent in your measurements. If you notice other changes, such as sleep quality or mental sharpness, then record these observations, too. Although these observations aren't quantitative, they can provide some additional evidence to you (and your partner) that your Male Infertility Hack is working. Be patient and keep excellent records. It may take a few weeks before you see significant results, so stick with your Hack strategy and keep recording your observations. For dietary changes to be effective, you will need to wait for your blood cells to turnover (be replaced). If your pre-Hack diet was inducing the ROS response in your blood cells, then it will take at least one week to replace your blood cells with healthy blood cells and your new Hack diet may prevent the ROS response. If you observe a marked difference in your Oxidative Stress level and sperm health, then you know the next test! Just maintain your new lifestyle and keep trying. You'll still be able to use the Urine Oxidative Stress Test kit to monitor your Oxidative Stress. If your still having difficulty despite a minimal Oxidative Stress level (and improved sperm health), then consult with your physician. There may be a different medical reason that warrants an investigation by your physician or your partner's physician. Use this Hack kit to rule out the possibility that **your** health is causing the problem.

Share Your Hack Results

This is where digitally recording your Male Infertility Hack information will come in handy, since it will be easier to compile these results and give people the best information available to Hack Male Infertility. Share your Hack Results on your own Blog or Social Media outlet. If you were successful in Hacking Male Infertility and improving your Sperm's Count and Health, then I'm sure your physician, family, and friends will want to learn more about it. If enough folks start Hacking Male Infertility with some success, then I will be happy to organize and report our group's results to the public.

Conclusion

This book is not the final word on Male Infertility with research reports streaming in every day. I'll keep reviewing the latest research and providing posts on my blog, so stop by and subscribe to receive the latest news. If you enjoy my book and found it helpful, then please consider reviewing it and sharing it.

Additional Information

Review My Book

If you enjoyed my book and used the Hack strategy with success, then please provide a review on Amazon or my website. If you're not comfortable providing a review of my book, then you can always send me a message through my blog site: http://hemagnosis.com/blog/wp/

BLOS World™ Store

If you're looking for recommendations on individual products or Hack kits, then stop by the BLOS World™ Store:

http://hemagnosis.com/blog/wp/shop/

BLOS Research

All proceeds from this book will be used to promote BLOS Research. **HemaGnosis** is currently developing a new blood test (BLOS#) for directly measuring the level of BLOS, which will be much more affordable compared to the flow cytometry method.